WEIGHT LOSS

THE EASIEST 3 STEPS TO WEIGHT LOSS FAST

CONTENTS

INTRODUCTION

Obesity and overweight in the United States. The number of obese Americans has increased at an alarming rate, especially over the past few years, to the point that the number of Americans today is overweight compared to normal weight. In fact, more than 60 percent of Americans are now overweight, with more than thirty percent of the population obese (for example, overweight by more than 20-30 percent of the recommended weight). These figures describe the tragic state of public health. Weight gain increases the risk of serious illness. A very large (and growing) proportion of citizens is at increased risk of serious chronic diseases and face the possibility of premature disability or death due to overweight. At the same time, the entire society is struggling under the burden of the resulting increase in health care costs.

For me, I have suffered from obesity for most of my life. I know the difficulties and problems of people who are obese, and like any person who is obese I have not been satisfied with myself. I tried to get rid of the extra weight. I followed many programs that claim that they can Make you thinner, and many more ways, but I did not benefit from them, sometimes we try so hard to find some answers to our questions, In the end, we discover that answer was always been in front of us, I got rid of obesity two years ago and this by following very simple steps, just don't give up and don't look back because you are not going that way.

This book concerns weight loss, an issue perpetually on many people's minds. Most everyone wants to be slim and toned. The following pages review the causes of weight gain, as well as the reasons why people devote the effort to reduce their weight to the recommended levels. Having provided motivation for a weight loss, we conclude with a survey of weight loss methods, and suggestions for achieving permanent healthy weight loss. Everyone's different, and no one diet is right for all. This book will help you to find a diet plan that works for you. Get started now by turning the page.

PART ONE
OBESITY

Obesity is a medical condition in which excess body fat accumulates to an extent that is a serious risk to health. Generally, People are considered obese when their body mass index, is over30 kg/m2, the range 25–30 kg/m2 is defined as overweight. The World Health Organization (WHO) has defined overweight thresholds, corresponding to a BMI between 25 and 30 kg / m².

BMI is measurement obtained by dividing a person's weight by the square of the person's height,

In 1997 obesity has been recognized as chronic disease by world health organization (WHO), This is due to the fact that obesity has become public health problem in developed countries.

Obesity increases the likelihood of serious illness, some of which may lead to paralysis or death. Like Type 2 diabetes, osteoporosis, cancer, and obstructive sleep apnea.

In the US, about 40 percent of adults (or 93.3 million people) are obese, according to the centers for disease control and prevention (CDC).

the world have been rising since 1975, the rate of obesity Some studies have shown that obesity rates around worldwide has tripled, and now more than 650 million people are obese, according to WHO estimates.

CHAPTER 1

WHY SHOULD YOU WORRY ABOUT OBESITY?

Generally, obesity is caused by moving too little and eating too much. If you consume high amounts of energy (fat and sugars), but don't burn off the energy through exercise and physical activity, much of the surplus energy will be stored by the body as fat.

Obesity can be dangerous to your body's health. Obese people are the most vulnerable to other diseases.

These diseases may lead to lower quality of health in people. In some cases, this can lead to disability or premature death.

CLORIES

Calories is a unit to measure the thermal energy needed by the body to do its work normally, by burning food. Man needs energy to do his basic functions of life, and this energy is the first source of food and oxygen that we breathe. Foods vary in the amount of energy they produce on the three essential elements of food: carbohydrates, proteins and fats.

mans needs about 2,500 calories a day to maintain a healthy weight, women need about 2,000 calories a day.

This value is not fixed. Different according to factors such as age, length and sex

This amount of calories may seem high, but it is easily accessible if you are eating certain types of food. For example, eating a large size hamburger, fries and milk can consume 1500 calories - and this is just one meal.

CHAPTER 2

MOST DANGEROUS DISEASES CAUSE BY OBESITY

1. Diabetes

The main cause of type 2 diabetes in general is obesity. People influenced by obesity or severe obesity are about 10 times more likely to have type 2 diabetes, Type 2 diabetes can nearly double the risk of death. Type 2 diabetes can lead to:

- Amputations

- Heart disease

- Stroke

- Blindness

- Kidney disease

- High blood pressure

- Circulatory and nerve defects

- Hard-to-heal infections

- Impotence

- And more

2. Hypertension

Obesity is a main risk factor for high blood pressure (also known as "hypertension").About 3 out of 4 hypertension cases are related to obesity. Hypertension increases the risk of other diseases. These include coronary heart disease, congestive heart failure, stroke, and kidney disease.

3. Heart Disease

Heart disease kills about 650,000 people every year in the United States. The American Heart Association considers obesity a primary risk factor for heart disease. Manny studies show that the risk for heart disease increases with obesity. People with severe obesity are facing higher risk for coronary artery disease. This means they have a higher risk of a heart attack than people who are not obese.

Obesity increases your risk of heart failure. Severe obesity is associated with irregular heartbeats (arrhythmias). However, some excess weight can protect you against dying from heart failure after the diagnosis is made.

4. Respiratory Disorders

People with obesity have reduced lung capacity. People who are more likely to have respiratory infections. They are more likely to have asthma and many other respiratory disorders. Asthma has been shown to be tow to three times more common among people with obesity.

More than half of those affected by obesity (around 50%-60%) obstructive sleep apnea In cases of severe obesity, this figure is around 90 percent). Obstructive sleep apnea is a serious breathing disorder. Obstructive sleep apnea occurs when excess fat in the neck, throat, and tongue block air passageways during sleep. This blockage cause apnea, which means a person stops breathing for a time. A person with obstructive sleep apnea may have hundreds of apnea episodes each night. Apnea episodes reduce the amount of oxygen in a person blood.

Obstructive sleep apnea may lead to high blood pressure, pulmonary hypertension, and heart failure. Obstructive sleep apnea can cause sudden cardiac death and stroke. Because of apnea episodes interrupt the normal sleep cycle, you may not reach restful sleep. This can lead to fatigue and drowsiness. If untreated, this drowsiness may raise your risk of vehicle accidents.

5. Cancer

Cancer affects more than half a million lives per year in the US alone. Obesity is believed to cause up to 100,000 cancer deaths per year. As body mass index increases, so does your risk of cancer and death from cancer. These cancers include:

- Endometrial cancer
- Cervical cancer
- Ovarian cancer
- Postmenopausal breast cancer
- Colorectal cancer
- Esophageal cancer
- Pancreatic cancer
- Gallbladder cancer
- Liver cancer
- Kidney cancer
- Thyroid cancer
- Prostate cancer
- Non-Hodgkin's lymphoma
- Multiple myeloma
- Leukemia

these people with severe obesity the death rate increases for all types of cancer. The death rate is 53 percent higher for men and 62 percent higher for women.

6. Cerebrovascular Disease and Stroke

Obesity causes a strain on your whole circulatory system. This strain increases your risk for stroke. Obesity can lead to other stroke risk factors. Stroke risk factors include heart disease, metabolic syndrome, hypertension, lipid abnormalities, type 2 diabetes and obstructive sleep apnea and more.

7. Gastro esophageal Reflux Disease

Gastro esophageal Reflux Disease (GERD) causes stomach acid or intestinal secretions to leak into your esophagus. Common Gastro esophageal Reflux Disease symptoms include heartburn, "indigestion", throwing up food, coughing (especially at night), hoarseness, and belching. Between 10% and 20 % of the general population experience GERD symptoms regularly.

Obesity has been associated with higher risk of Gastro esophageal Reflux Disease, erosive esophagitis and rarely, esophageal cancer (adenocarcinoma).

8. Bone/Joint Damage and Accidents

Obesity, in particular severe obesity, contributes to a number of joint and Bone issues. These issues can increase the risk for personal injury and accident. Bone and joint issues can include:

- Joint diseases (osteoarthritis, gout)

- Disc herniation

- Spinal disorders

- Back pain

- Pseudo tumor cerebra, a condition associated with disorientation, headache, and visual impairment.

PART TWO
CAUSES OF OBESITY

Obesity doesn't happen overnight. Obesity develops gradually over time, as a result of poor diet and lifestyle choices and other factors such as:

CHAPTER 3

1. Poor diet

• **Eating Large Amounts Of Processed Or Fast Food** that's high in fat and sugar, There are four basic reasons why fast food is linked to obesity.

Unhealthy Ingredients

Most of the fast food contains a large amount of sugar, carb and fats and less minerals and vitamins. This means that you are taking in large amount of unhealthy calories which leads to weight gain and ultimately obesity. Most of the fast foods have exceeding levels of fats and sugars which are directly associated with increasing weight.

Larger Portions

The unhealthy ingredients of the fast food are further aggravated with increased portion sizes which have grown with the average body weight of a person from the 70s to date. While the portions have become large now, the person will still eat the complete meal regardless of feeling full or not. This means that people are eating bigger portions of junk food leading to obesity.

Lower Cost

One of the main reasons people can't stop eating fast food is the low costs it is available in. As per a research conducted by the University of Washington, a diet containing 2000 calories of fast food costs much less than a diet with 2000 calories of healthy food. This makes it more affordable than going for healthy food and is a major cause of obesity in lower-income classes.

Convenience

Fast food restaurants offer convenience. You can always find one in close proximity of your home and can also get food easily delivered to your place. And this makes it a convenient option than making food at home using healthier ingredients.

Some studies have shown, the consumption of fast food has increased over the past four decades at an alarming rate. This increased calorie intake is a leading cause of obesity in USA. If it is not controlled, health issues are going to rise in the coming years as more people will become obese eating unhealthy food.

• **Drinking too much alcohol** – alcohol contains a lot of calories, and these people who drink heavily are often overweight.

Obesity and alcoholism may be more related than we realize. Both conditions are occasioned by periods of loss of control, whether that loss of control is the result of a moment of personal weakness, environment or the genetics. People with these conditions spend a lot of time preoccupied with managing their addiction, whether it is feeling guilty, struggling to maintain control or planning how and when they will next access alcohol or food. Both conditions can grow progressively worse and both, taken to an extreme, can be fatal.

Part of what makes obesity and alcoholism alike is the way the tools of the disease, ethanol and food, work on the brain. Ethanol stimulates reward centers in the brain in much the same way sugar, fat and salt do. Because of this, people who have predisposition to over-drinking may also have a predisposition to overeating."

Alcohol and Weight-loss

Some people said that drinking alcohol increases appetite, and so can lead to overeating and weight gain. Ethanol, the kind of alcohol in alcoholic drinks, and fat from foods have approximately the same amount of calories (body fat); but people with alcoholism tend not to be affected by obesity, mainly because they are often malnourished, having replaced a portion of their food calories with alcohol calories. Some turn to alcohol, just as others turn to drugs or cigarettes, as a way to replace the comfort they find in food.

A 2005 study looked at these people who drank alcoholic drinks regularly. It showed that people who drank the smallest amount (one drink per day) with the greatest frequency (four to seven days per week) had a lower body mass index than those who drank more infrequently, but in larger amounts. While we can't claim a effect and causes from the results, they may show a relationship between over-drinking and overeating.

In addition, a small study of 15 men who added two glasses of red wine to their evening meal every day for 12 weeks, showed no measured effect on the weight, body fat (calorie) intake of the men involved. While both studies suggest that moderate drinking (one to two drinks per day) is not associated with higher body mass index, it is not a good idea for those interested in losing weight to turn alcohol as a replacement for food. This trade-off is an unhealthy one, and those people who interested in losing weight would be better off focusing on their current condition instead of trading one for another.

A Growing Link between Alcoholism and Obesity

Researchers at the Washington University School of Medicine. Louis published one of the most important studies done regarding the link between alcoholism and obesity in early 2011. They looked at data of two large alcoholism surveys. The first one, the National Longitudinal Alcohol Epidemiologic Survey, was conducted in 1991-1992. And the second, the National Epidemiologic Survey on Alcohol and Related

Conditions, was conducted in 2001-2002. In all, 90,000 people took part in the two surveys.

After contro ling for other factors, the researchers found that in the more recent survey, people with a family history of alcoholism had a greater chance to get obesity. For women, who had a 48 percent greater chance, this was especially true. One possible explanation is that in trying to avoid the alcoholic behaviors observed in their families, people try to replace alcohol with a different addiction.

What surprised researchers, was that there was no link between obesity and a family history of alcoholism in the first survey. The fact that the link strengthened as much as it did in the relatively short amount of time between the two surveys suggests that environmental factors (the increased prevalence of fatty the increase in sedentary times, sugary and salty foods in grocery stores and restaurants; and the reduced access to opportunities for activity) are involved. In short, a genetic risk may be subdued in a world that makes maintaining one's weight a relatively straightforward task. But, change the environment to make unhealthy eating easier and being active harder, and that, will make the problem apparent.

The researchers comments in their publication in the Archives of Psychiatry are telling. They focused on some changes to our food environment, suggesting that obesity may be rising in "individuals vulnerable to addiction. This could be specifically the result of a changing food environment and the increased availability of highly palatable foods."

Overlapping Brain Pathways

Neuroscientists are finding similarities in the pathways that lead to dependence and excessive eating on alcohol and other drugs. Both alcohol and obesity addiction have been linked to the brain's reward system. Overconsumption can trigger a gradual increase in the reward threshold, requiring more palatable high-fat food or reinforcing alcohol to satisfy cravings.

The National Institutes of Health researchers have recently found that exposure to high-fat foods can trigger addictive responses in animals and cause obesity. Dr. Nora Volkow, the director of the National Institute (NI) for Drug Abuse, said, "Addiction and obesity are two of the most challenging health problems in the US.

This research opens the door for us to apply some of the knowledge we have gathered about addiction to the study of obesity and overeating ."

Likewise, researchers have recently shown that a brain protein named neuropeptide-Y regulates alcohol use, as well as appetite and food consumption. According to Dr. Todd Thiele, "Every day we are learning more about how drinking and eating are inextricably linked at the physiologic level. These physiologic commonalities help to explain why the behaviors of excessive alcohol consumption and excessive food intake share so much similarities."

• **Eating larger portions than you need** – you may be encouraged to eat too much if your friends or relatives are also eating large portions, and more food means more calories which if not burned become to fat.

• **Drinking too many sugary drinks** — Sugary drinks have frequently been cited as a seemingly innocuous, easily available product with a harmful potential when it comes to preserving our health. A study published last year, for example, showed that the consumption of sugar-sweetened beverages is linked to the onset of metabolic diseases.

Researchers from multiple institutions across the globe — including the Special Institute for Nutrition in Salzburg and Preventive Cardiology, Austria, the Geneva University Hospitals in Switzerland, and the University of Navarra in Spain — have teamed up to analyze recent studies targeting the potential link between sugary drink and obesity.

"The evidence base linking with overweight and obesity in adults and children's has grown in the past 3 years, The researchers looked at 20 studies addressing the link between obesity and SSBs in children (17 prospective and three randomized controlled trials), and also 10 studies investigating this link between obesity and SSBs in the case of adults (nine prospective and one randomized controlled trial).

Of all the studies, 93 percent concluded that there was a "positive association" between the onset of overweight or obesity and the consumption of sugary drinks in both children and adults.

Just one prospective cohort study found no link between SSBs and excess weight in the case of children.

• **Comfort eating** – if you feel depressed or you have low self-esteem, you may eat to make yourself feel better Unhealthy eating habits tend to run in families.

CHAPTER 4

2. Lack of physical activity

Lack of physical activity is another important factor that causes to obesity. Most people have jobs that involve sitting at a desk for most of the day. They also rely on their cars, rather than cycling or walking.

For relaxation, many people tend to watch TV, play computer games or browse the internet, and rarely take regular exercise.

If you're not active enough, you are not using the energy provided by the food you eat, and the extra energy you consume is stored by the body as fat.

The Department of Health recommends that adults do at least 150 minutes of moderated intensity aerobic activity, such as fast walking or cycling, every week. This does not need to be done at once, but can be broken down into smaller periods. For example, you could exercise for 30 minutes to 45 minutes a day for five days a week.

CHAPTER 5

3. GENETIC

If you're obese and trying to lose weight, maybe you need to do more exercise then this. It may help you to start off slowly and gradually increase the amount of exercise you do each week.

Some people claim that there is no point in trying to lose weight "because it is in my genes" or "in my family".

While there are some genetic cases that can cause obesity which is very rare, there is no reason why most people lose weight.

There is a possibility that genetic traits inherited from your parents - such as having a large appetite - make weight loss more difficult perhaps, but it certainly does not make it impossible.

In many cases, obesity is linked more to environmental factors, such as bad eating habits that have been learned during childhood, or "physical inactivity".

CHAPTER 6

4. Medical reasons

There are some rare cases, basic medical conditions may contribute to weight gain. These include:

• an under active thyroid gland (hypothyroidism) – where your thyroid gland doesn't produce enough hormones.

• Cushing's syndrome – a rare disorder that causes the overproduction of steroid hormones.

However, if conditions such as these are properly treated and diagnosed, they should pose less of a barrier to weight loss.

Certain medicines, including some corticosteroid, medications for epilepsy and diabetes, and some medications used to treat mental illness – including antidepressants and medicines for schizophrenia – can contribute to weight gain.

Weight gain can be a side effect of stopping smoking.

PART THREE
WEIGHT LOSS

Weight Loss in the fields of medicine, health and fitness means any loss of mass body mass, because of the loss of liquids or body fat or fatty tissues and / or the body of the body (the body mass without fat), especially: mixed breeding bones, the muscles, thesis, and other massacles. Weight is not intertwined: Caused by malnutrition or campaign, or the creation of a genital or gesture, the objective of the sports or the dissolution of the sports "," The universal excuse, the unlearning. The extent of the diligent Well is called a solic, and the loss of the deliberate weight is called the storm.

Weight gain is usually associated with excessive consumption of fats, sugars and refined carbohydrates in general as well as alcohol. Depression, stress and boredom may also contribute to weight gain, in which case people are advised to seek medical help. A study in 2010 suggests that dieters who sleep all night are more likely to lose twice as much fat as dieters who are deprived of sleep at night.

Most dieters regain their long-term weight.

According to the American Food Guidelines, people who reach a healthy weight do so successfully by taking care to consume enough calories to meet their needs and exercise. According to the US Food and Drug Administration, healthy people seeking to maintain their weight should consume 2,000 calories at 8.4 megawatts per day.

There are many ways to lose weight fast.

However, most of them will make you unsatisfied and hungry‹ then hunger will cause you to give up on these plans quickly.

The plan outlined here will:

- Reduce your appetite significantly.
- Make you lose a lot of weight fast and without hunger.
- Improve your metabolic health.

3 STEPS TO WEIGHT LOSS FAST

CHAPTER 7

1. Cut Back on Sugars and Starches

The most important part is to cut back on sugars and carbs.

When you do, hunger levels go down and this will make you eat much less calories.

Now instead of burning carbohydrates to get energy, your body starts to burn stored fat to get the energy that he need.

Another benefit of cutting carbs is that it lowers insulin levels causing your water out of your body.". This reduces bloat and unnecessary water weight.

It is not uncommon to lose up to 10 pounds or more in the first week of eating this way, both body fat and water weight.

Cut off carbohydrates and you will begin to eat less calories automatically and without hunger.

Simply put, cutting carbohydrates makes you lose weight automatically.

SUMMARY

Removing starches (carbs) and sugars from your diet will reduce your appetite, lower your insulin levels and make you lose weight without hunger.

CHAPTER 8

2. Eat Protein, Fat and Vegetables

Each one of your daily meals should include a fat source, protein source and low-carb vegetables.

If you build your meals this way you will automatically enter the amount of carbohydrates in the recommended range of 20 to 50 grams per day.

Protein Sources

1. Eggs

35% of calories in a whole egg. 1 large egg has 6g of protein, with 78 calories.

2. Almonds

13% of calories. 6g per ounce (28 g), with 161 calories.

3. Chicken Breast

80% of calories. 1 roasted chicken breast without skin contains 53 g, with 284 calories.

4. Oats

5% of calories. Half a cup of raw oats has 13 g, with 303 calories.

5. Cottage Cheese

59% of calories. A cup (226 g) of cottage cheese with 2% fat contains 27 g of protein, with 194 calories.

6. Greek Yogurt

Non-fat Greek, 48% of calories. One 6-ounce (170 g) container has 17 g of protein, with only 100 calories.

7. Milk

21% of calories. 1 cup of milk contains 8 g of protein, with 149 calories.

8. Broccoli

20% of calories. 1 cup (96 grams) of chopped broccoli has 3 g of protein, with only 31 calories.

9. Lean Beef

53% of calories. One 3-ounce (85 g) serving of cooked beef with 10% fat contains 22 g of protein, with 184 calories.

10. Tuna

94% of calories, in tuna canned in water. A cup (154 g) contains 39 g of protein, with only 179 calories.

11. Quinoa

15% of calories. One cup (185 g) of cooked quinoa has 8 g, with 222 calories.

12. Whey Protein Supplements

Varies between brands. Can go over 90% of calories, with 20-50 g of protein per serving.

13. Lentils

27% of calories. 1 cup (198 g) of boiled lentils contains 18 g, with 230 calories.

14. Ezekiel Bread

20% of calories. 1 slice contains 4 g, with 80 calories.

15. Pumpkin Seeds

14% of calories. 1 ounce (28 g) has 5 g of protein, with 125 calories.

16. Turkey Breast

70% of calories. One 3-ounce (85 g) serving contains 24 g, with 146 calories.

17. Fish (All Types)

Highly variable. Salmon is 46% protein, with 19 g per 3-ounce (85 g) serving and only 175 calories.

18. Shrimp

90% of calories. A 3 ounce (85 g) serving contains 18 g, with only 84 calories.

19. Brussels Sprouts

17% of calories. Half a cup (78 g) contains 2 g of protein, with 28 calories.

20. Peanuts

16% of calories. One ounce (28 g) has 7 g, with 159 calories.

The importance of eating protein cannot be overstated.

This has been shown to boost metabolism about 70 to 100 calories per day.

Low-carb Vegetables source

Vegetables are low calories and rich in vitamins, minerals and other important nutrients.

In addition, many vegetables are low in carbs and high in fiber, making them best ideal for low-carb diets.

The definition of a low-carb diet varies widely. Most are under 150 g of carbs per day, and some go as low as 20 g per day.

Whether you're on a low-carb diet or not, eating more vegetables is a great idea.

1. Bell Peppers

One cup (149 g) of chopped red pepper contains 9 grams of carbs, 3 of which are fiber.

2. Broccoli

One cup (91 g) of raw broccoli contains 6 grams of carbs, 2 of which are fiber.

3. Asparagus

One cup (180 g) of cooked asparagus contains 8 grams of carbs, 4 of which are fiber. And it's a good source of vitamins A, C and K.

4. Mushrooms

one cup (70-g) serving of raw, white mushrooms contains just 2 grams of carbs, 1 of which is fiber.

5. Zucchini

One cup (124 g) of raw zucchini contains 4 grams of carbs, 1 of which is fiber. And it's a good source of vitamin C, providing 35% of the RDI per serving.

6. Spinach

One cup (180 g) of cooked spinach provides more than 10 times the RDI for vitamin K.

7. Avocados

one cup (150-g) serving of chopped avocados has 13 grams of carbs, 10 of which are fiber.

8. Cauliflower

One cup (100 g) of raw cauliflower contains 5 grams of carbs, 3 of which are fiber. And it's also high in vitamin K and provides 77% of the RDI for vitamin C.

9. Green Beans

one cup (125-g) serving of cooked green beans contains 10 grams of carbs, 4 of which are fiber.

10. Lettuce

One cup (47 g) of lettuce contains 2 grams of carbs, 1 of which is fiber.

11. Garlic

One clove (3 g) of garlic contains 1 gram of carbs, part of which is fiber.

12. Kale

One cup (67 g) of raw kale contains 7 grams of carbs, 1 of which is fiber. And it also provides an impressive 206% of the RDI for vitamin A and 134% of the RDI for vitamin C.

13. Cucumbers

One cup (104 g) of chopped cucumber contains 4 grams of carbs, less than 1 gram of which is fiber.

14. Brussels Sprouts

half cup (78 g) serving of cooked Brussels sprouts contains 6 grams of carbs, 2 of which are fiber.

15. Celery

one cup (101g) serving of chopped celery contains 3 grams of carbs, 2 of which are fiber. And it's a good source of vitamin K, providing 37% of the RDI.

16. Tomatoes

One cup (149 g) of cherry tomatoes contains 6 grams of carbs, 2 of which are fiber.

17. Radishes

One cup (116 g) of raw sliced radishes contains 4 grams of carbs, 2 of which are fiber.

18. Onions

A half cup (58 g) of sliced raw onions contains 6 grams of carbs, 1 of which is fiber.

19. Eggplant

A one-cup (99 g) serving of chopped, cooked eggplant contains 8 grams of carbs, 2 of which are fiber.

20. Cabbage

One cup (89 g) of chopped raw cabbage contains 5 grams of carbs, 3 of which are fiber.

Do not be afraid to add these low-carbohydrate vegetables to your meals. You can eat huge amounts of them without exceeding 30 to 50 net carbohydrates per day.

A diet that relies mostly on vegetables and meat contains all the vitamins, minerals and fiber you need to be healthy.

Olive oil coconut

oil avocado

oil butter

Eat 2–3 meals per day. in the afternoon you may feel hungry, you can add a 4th meal.

Don't be afraid of eating fat, as trying to do both low-fat and low-carb at the same time is a recipe for failure. It will make you abandon the plan.

CHAPTER 9
3. LIFT WEIGHTS

You don't need to exercise so hard to lose weight on this plan.

The best option is to exercise 3-4 times a week. Lift some weights and do not forget to warm up before exercise. And if you're new to the gym, ask a trainer for some advice.

lifting weights, will make you burn lots of calories and prevent your metabolism from slowing down, which is a common side effect of losing weight.

Some studies on low-carb diets show that you can even gain a bit of muscle while losing significant amounts of body fat.

If lifting weights is not an option for you, then doing some cardio workouts like walking, running, cycling or swimming will suffice.

CHAPTER 10

DAY OFF (optional)

You can take one day off per two weeks where you eat more carbs.

It is important to stick to healthy carb sources like rice, oats, potatoes, sweet potatoes, fruit, etc.

But only this one higher carb day — if you start doing it more often than once per two weeks you're not going to see much success on this plan.

If you must have a cheat meal then do it on this day.

Be aware that cheat meals or carb refeeds are NOT necessary, but they can boost some fat-burning hormones like thyroid hormones and leptin.

You will gain some weight during your refeed day, but most of it will be water weight and you will lose it again in the next 1–2 day so don't worry.

CHAPTER 11

HOW FAST YOU WILL LOST WEIGHT

When you have a significant amount of weight to drop or an imminent deadline, trying to shed unwanted pounds quickly is pretty tempting. Here's what you need to know in order to do effectively and safely!

If you have more to lose, you will lose more—initially. It's actually more useful to think of the weight you want to lose in terms of a percentage of your current weight, rather than thinking in number of pounds. "For most men, a weight loss goal of 10% to 15% is a reasonable place to start," says Nisha Basu, M.D., a primary care physician at Beth Israel Deaconess Medical Center. So for a man who weighs 225, that would be 24 to 34 pounds. For one who weighs 350, he's looking at 33 to 53 pounds—at least as a starting point. The bigger guy may also, drop more pounds in his first few weigh-ins. Pace of weight loss is variable. "In general, for those with more weight to lose, initial weight loss can happen more rapidly."

That first weigh-in may be dramatic. It's not uncommon to see that scale needle make a satisfying downtick within the first week or the second of changing your habits. "Generally the first week, most people can lose few pounds, which is mainly water weight," says Basu. Why? When you put your body at a calorie deficit (eat fewer calories than you burn), your body immediately goes to its ready-energy stores of glycogen (basically, a form of sugar) to make up the difference. In the process, water is released.

When the glycogen is depleted and the body figures out it needs another way to find fuel, that's when the actual weight loss begins.

Not all weight loss is equal. Aside from that tricky glycogen-fueled water weight, the body can burn both fat (yay!) and muscle (not-so-yay) as fuel. Not only that, burning fat for energy isn't nearly as easy at a cellular level as burning sugar… or protein (really not-so-yay). "Weight training and eating enough protein is key to not losing muscle mass. Increasing your muscle mass can help to weight loss. That's why strength training may actually be more important than cardio in supporting a weight loss plan.

There's a legit reason that pacing is key. You probably keep hearing about that whole 1-to-2 pound-per-week rule of thumb and think, I can do better than that!" but hear us—and the Harvard doctor—out. "Almost every time a patient loses a large amount of weight in a short time, like 10 pounds in a week, the patient will gain it all back and more. "Further, several studies have shown that this dieting is harmful to a person's long-term health." So basically, you may drop the lbs for the reunion, but you may be in a pickle to drop them again for the next one five years from now.

You should learn healthy eating habits and how to combine exercise and activities in your life. Because if you do not learn how to make real lifestyle changes, you will return to your old habits and ... know the rest. "In addition, metabolism slows down significantly in response to this type of Weight loss.

Everyone plateaus—and can persevere. So, unfortunately, you're stuck losing weight at a slow pace after all. An even more annoying reality check: Even that pace will inevitably stop. When a plateau happens, it could be that you've let some old bad habits crop back up. Or you may simply need to make some changes to what you've been doing, even though that exact plan was working so well mere weeks ago. Like for a person begins to weigh less, he needs fewer calories to support the new lower body weight. But by simply tweaking portion exercise (more) or size (smaller), you'll be back to losing in no time.

www.ingramcontent.com/pod-product-compliance
Lightning Source LLC
Chambersburg PA
CBHW050757290526
45792CB00008B/2226